Growing Up Grounded

Learning to cope with a parent who suffers from mental illness
An art-based workbook

By: Shelby Wynn, MS

Acknowledgements

To both of my parents, I wouldn't change a single thing about the conditions that I grew up in. Without those trials and tribulations (don't worry you both had your moments), I would never have grown up to be who I am today, and I may never have stumbled upon the field of art therapy. Even throughout the not so great times, we managed to all stick together and stay close. To my little brother Camren, who was always there to listen to my heartaches and frustrations, I just had to get up the courage to go into that stinky room! Without having you to come home to every night, I am not sure that I would have made it through the majority of graduate school. And, finally, to the faculty that helped me get to where I am - writing books for God's sake - you all have guided me through a very fragile time in my life and helped me figure out a way to use those experiences. The knowledge that I gained from the art therapy program will hopefully fill a very desperate hole in adolescent literature.

Table of Contents

Note From the Author   1

Chapter One   2
I'm In A Situation

Chapter Two   8
There is Help For My Situation

Chapter Three   14
I Make A Commitment To Follow All Suggestions

Chapter Four   20
Who Am I?

Chapter Five   26
I Will Share Who I Am With Someone Else

Chapter Six   32
I See Things About Myself That I Would Like To Change

Chapter Seven   38
I Start Trying To Change What I Can

Chapter Eight   44
I Make A List Of People Who I Have Mistreated Or Whom I Have Ill Feelings Towards

Chapter Nine   50
If Possible, I Mend Things With These People So That I Can Get Rid Of My Bad Feelings

Chapter Ten   56
I Look At Me Daily. How Am I Doing: Physically, Mentally, Emotionally, And Spiritually

Chapter Eleven   62
I Continue To Grow As A Human Being Daily

Chapter Twelve   68
I Try To Help Others In My Situation, And To Practice What I Have Learned In All Areas Of My Life

Author Biography   74

A List of Resources   75

In Case You Needed Proof:

This workbook was designed to engage adolescents in strategies and activities to foster coping skills. These skills will be cultivated through developmentally appropriate art processes, media, and directives that may promote self-awareness, coping, and/or serve as a tool in art therapy sessions in which the work may be discussed with an art therapist. An adolescent living with a parent who is suffering from a mental illness often begin to show signs of psychopathology themselves early in development (Bartsch et al., 2014; Berg-Nielsen & Wichstrom, 2012; Van Loon, Van de Ven, Van Doesum, Witteman, & Hosman, 2013).

A mental disorder is a pattern of thoughts and/or behavior that is characterized by a significant disturbance in an individual's daily life. This condition may affect the individual's cognition and emotional regulation, or display a disturbance in the biological, psychological, or developmental processes of mental functioning (American Psychiatric Association, 2013). In most cases, it is up to the children to care for their mentally ill parent(s) (Aldridge & Sharpe, 2009). These children have been known to suffer from anxiety and depression (Stoeckel & Weissbrod, 2014; Ola, Suren, & Ani, 2015), as well as behavioral problems, which likely stem from the strained parenting style (Wansink et al., 2015). The children themselves are also at a greater risk for developing guilt or anger in response to coping with their parent's mental illness, Post Traumatic Stress Disorder (PTSD), developmental delays, and many other mental, physical, and emotional disabilities (Mental health of America of Hawaii, n.d.).

Parents may find it difficult to be responsive to their child; they may be withdrawn with a potential for neglect and abuse (Mental Health America of Hawaii, n.d.). Adolescents, because of their developing life stage, may generally lack sufficient coping skills to adequately propel themselves through the stressful experience of having a parent with mental illness. The Al-Anon and Ala-Teen groups have been using the 12-steps to aid in building the coping skills of the families and teens effected by a family member battling an addiction (Welcome to Al-Anon Family Groups, 2015). The 12-step is used as a guide because it is a structured approach and seems to be developmentally appropriate for adolescents who are capable of increasing autonomy and independence (self-help) and who still require guidance (structure of 12-steps). Research shows that art making can reduce an individual's stress levels and states of anxiety. An art-based workbook may serve as a bridge to connect adolescents with the coping skills and resources they may need to decrease anxiety, depression, and promote healing while living with a parent who suffers from mental illness. (Lagaca-Saguin et al, 2012).

A Note From the Author:

Obviously, there is something going on in your family that is causing you stress, or you wouldn't have picked up this book. Maybe your parent or caregiver has been recently diagnosed with a mental illness, or you have always felt that something was up. First of all, don't worry, you are not alone. Do you think I would be writing this book if you were? Of all the adults diagnosed (or not) with a mental illness, the majority of them are parents and little to no attention is paid to their children and how this diagnosis also affects their children. I would like to take you through twelve chapters, helping you as the child, to cope with your current family situation. Allow me to take you on a creative journey that I wish I were exposed to as a child of a parent with a mental illness.

Each chapter will focus on a certain coping skill that may help you live a better life at home. You will begin each chapter assessing where you think you are with the current topic at that very moment. Do you think you have a pretty good grasp on a chapter's topic? Maybe you need some work, or you know for sure that you could use some help with that chapter? From there, you will be asked to explore through art and writing, some pretty difficult topics at times. Do not feel like you have to rush through each chapter. Sometimes, you may feel the need to spend a few days or even weeks, and that is encouraged. Learning to overcome the obstacle is okay! This book is for you and only you – go at your own pace. At the end of the chapter, you will be asked to reflect through art and/or writing, what you have learned and how you can implement the skill into your daily life.

You may notice that each chapter is labeled "Step _____". This is because each chapter is modified from a list of steps from the 12 Steps for Teens. Usually, when people hear about 12 Step programs, they immediately think Alcoholics Anonymous, but there are many different groups. There are many different programs for many different issues that people face in life every day. The steps will allow you to have a guideline to follow and a clear goal set for you at the end. It always seems to help me more in life if I have something visible to work towards! These pages will be filled with sometimes very private thoughts and images. It is up to you whether you want to show anyone. Be honest with yourself and really think about each of the chapters and how they could improve your situation. You can do this...
I am rooting for you!

Oh, I almost forgot! You do not need to be an artist for this workbook to help you. Art is unique to everyone and is a great way to get your thoughts and feelings out when it comes to things that you may not be ready to talk about aloud yet. As for art supplies, you can use anything you have on hand at the moment. Are there still coffee grounds from this morning's coffee? Those could make a really neat statement on one of these pages. Art can be as simple as pencils and markers, or as complex as coffee grounds and watercolors.

"Every child is an artist. The problem is how to remain
an artist once we grow up"
Pablo Picasso

Step One

I'm in a Situation

I admit that I am powerless over my situation and that my life has become unmanageable.

Honesty

This may be one of the most challenging steps that you will take while working through this book. Maybe you are sixteen, ten, or even eight years old and you have spent the majority of your life trying to convince yourself that what is going on at home is normal. The most important thing for you to realize is that, yes, this is real, and, no, it is NOT your fault. I can promise you that you are not the only one experiencing a home life that is less than perfect. Even during my own situation, I tried to rationalize it and say, "Who am I to complain when some kids have it so much worse?" Let me tell you something - those kids are not you and you are fully allowed to acknowledge that something isn't right in your home life.

Writing Directive

Family Secret's: Its time to get honest with yourself... Pretend you are writing a letter to a younger you. What would you tell them about your family as of today? What is so challenging that you have turned to this book for help?

_____
_____
_____
_____
_____
_____
_____
_____
_____
_____
_____
_____
_____
_____
_____
_____
_____
_____
_____
_____
_____
_____

*" I think the most important thing you can do to be a real person -
is to be honest with yourself."
Mike Dirnt*

Art Space

Draw a road map showing how the journey of your life has been affected by your family secret

Process What You Have Learned

Use this space to reflect on your thoughts, feelings, and ideas about what has come up for you while working through this chapter:

_____
_____
_____
_____
_____
_____
_____
_____
_____
_____
_____
_____
_____
_____
_____
_____
_____
_____
_____
_____
_____
_____
_____
_____
_____

Closing Artwork

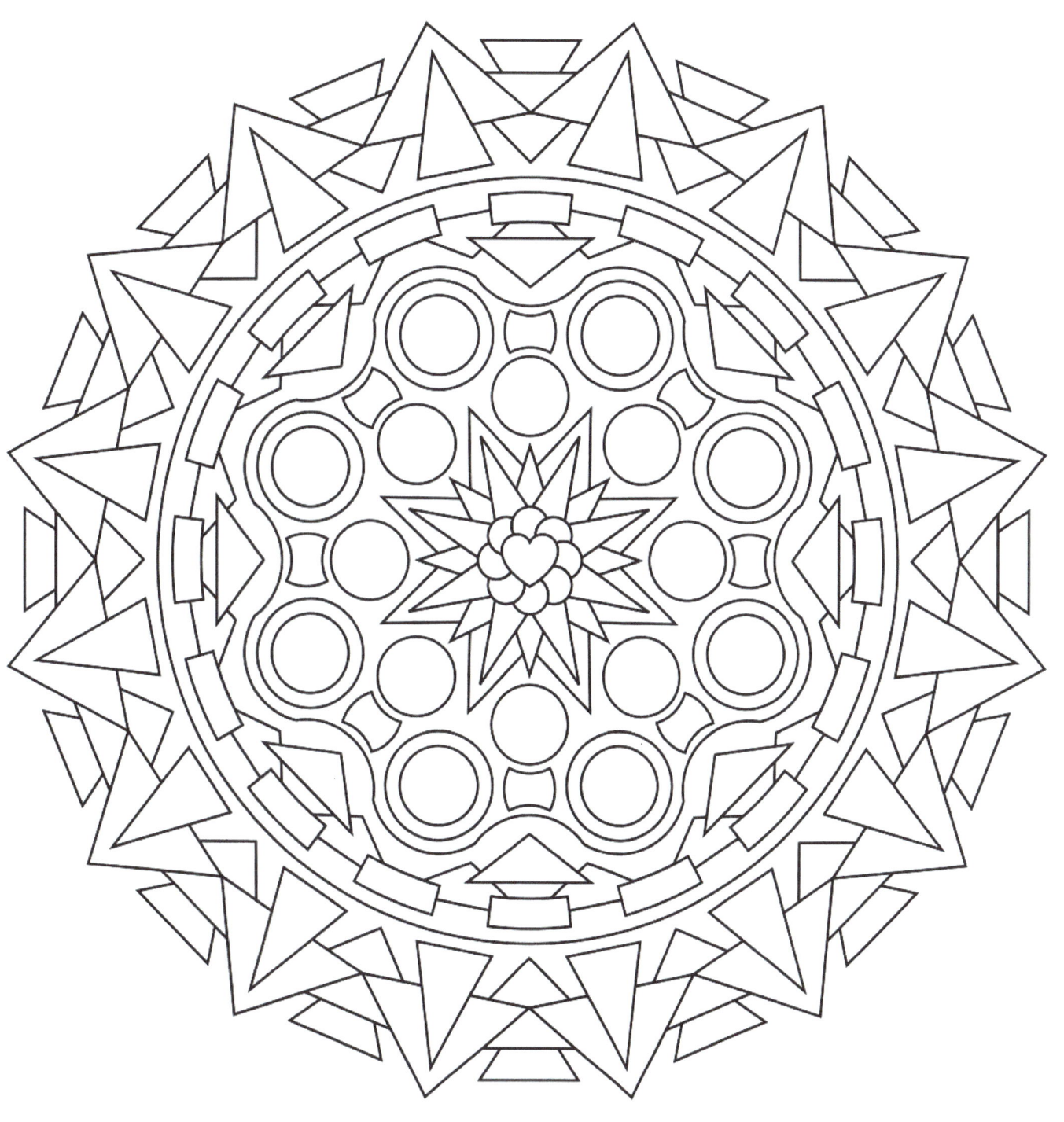

Step Two

There's help for my situation

I have come to believe that something greater than myself could restore me to balance

Hope

Hope is something that you must have in order to get anywhere in life. If you don't hope and you don't believe that there is a chance your situation can get better, there is no way that it will. Sometimes the saying 'Fake It Till You Make It" is the only real option you have until you convince yourself that there is a light at the end of the tunnel. I spent many, many years sad and depressed because I had convinced myself that no matter what I did, nothing was every going to get better. I came up with every excuse in the book for why I deserved a life of distress with my parents. No one deserves the feelings that you are feeling.

Writing Directive

Imagine you go to sleep tonight and when you wake up in the morning everything is better. Describe what it would be like when you awake and everything is better...was there a certain person, event, or thing that helped it to turn around?

_____
_____
_____
_____
_____
_____
_____
_____
_____
_____
_____
_____
_____
_____
_____
_____
_____
_____
_____
_____
_____
_____
_____

"Let your hopes, not your hurts, shape your future."
Robert H. Shuller

Art Space

Create an image that shows how it would look if everthing in your life was the way you wanted it to be.

Process What You Have Learned

Use this space to reflect on your thoughts, feelings, and ideas about what has come up for you while working through this chapter:

_____
_____
_____
_____
_____
_____
_____
_____
_____
_____
_____
_____
_____
_____
_____
_____
_____
_____
_____
_____
_____
_____

Closing Artwork

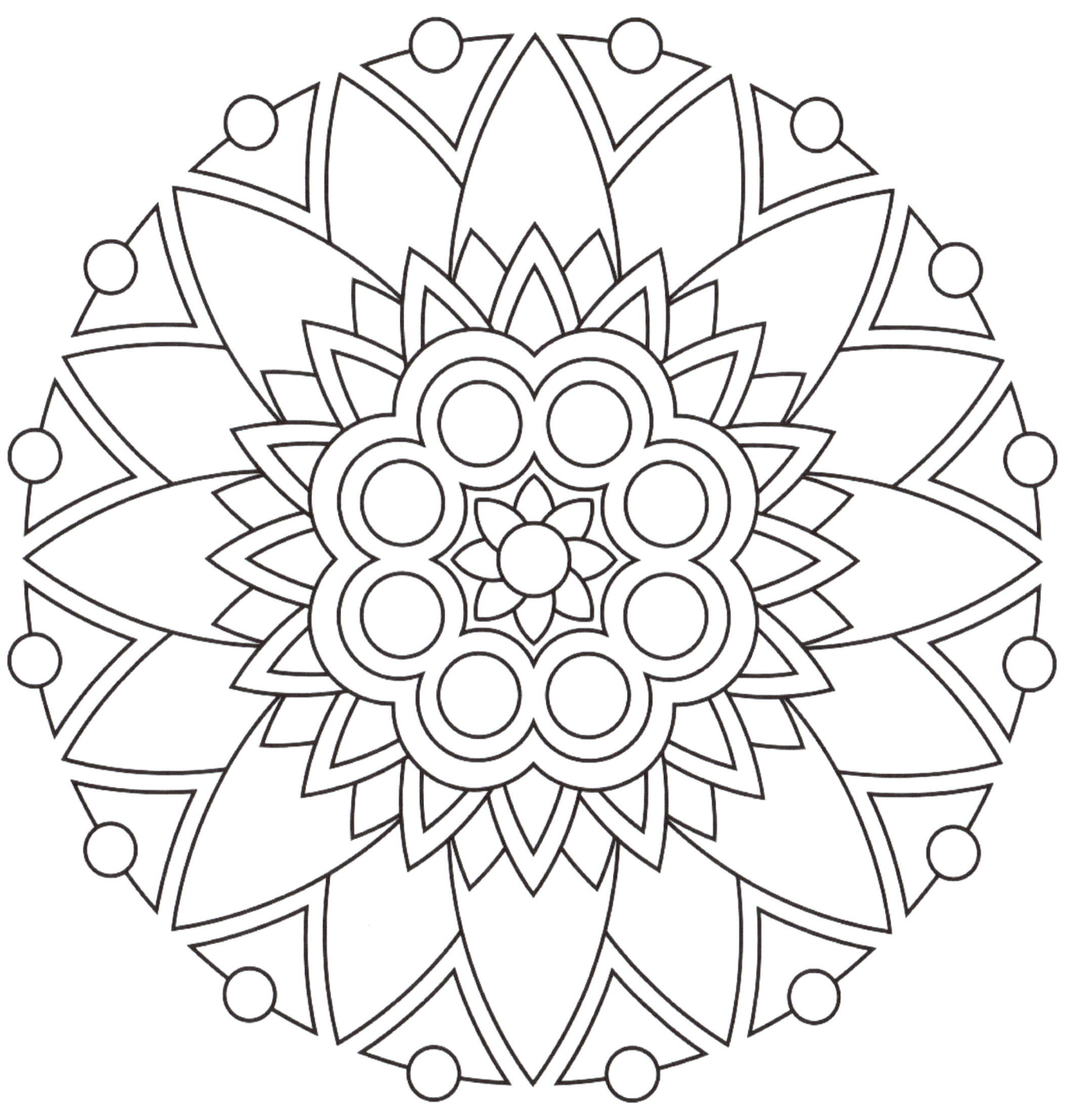

Step Three

I will make a commitment

I made a decision to turn my will and my life over to the care and help of someone else

Trust

Trust... How do you learn to trust someone when you have never had anyone to fully count on in life? Maybe I shouldn't assume that you don't have someone special to trust. Is it possible that you have just never considered certain people as willing to help you? Thinking back on my childhood and teenage years, I now see all of the people that would have dropped everything to help me or even given me the chance to get some things off my chest. A trusted person can be someone who you least expect: your 8th grade biology teacher, your best friend's mom, maybe even someone in your own extended family (if it is someone in your family, make sure that they are able to be unbiased and not take sides).

Writing Directive

Who is someone that you trust? What characteristics make them a trustworthy person? If you do not feel that you trust anyone, can you explain why?

"I'll lean on you and you lean on me and we'll be okay."
Dave Matthews

Art Space

Draw a portrait or symbol of the person that you trust more than anyone else.
List their positive qualities too!

Process What You Have Learned

Use this space to reflect on your thoughts, feelings, and ideas about what has come up for you while working through this chapter:

_____
_____
_____
_____
_____
_____
_____
_____
_____
_____
_____
_____
_____
_____
_____
_____
_____
_____
_____
_____
_____
_____
_____
_____

Closing Artwork

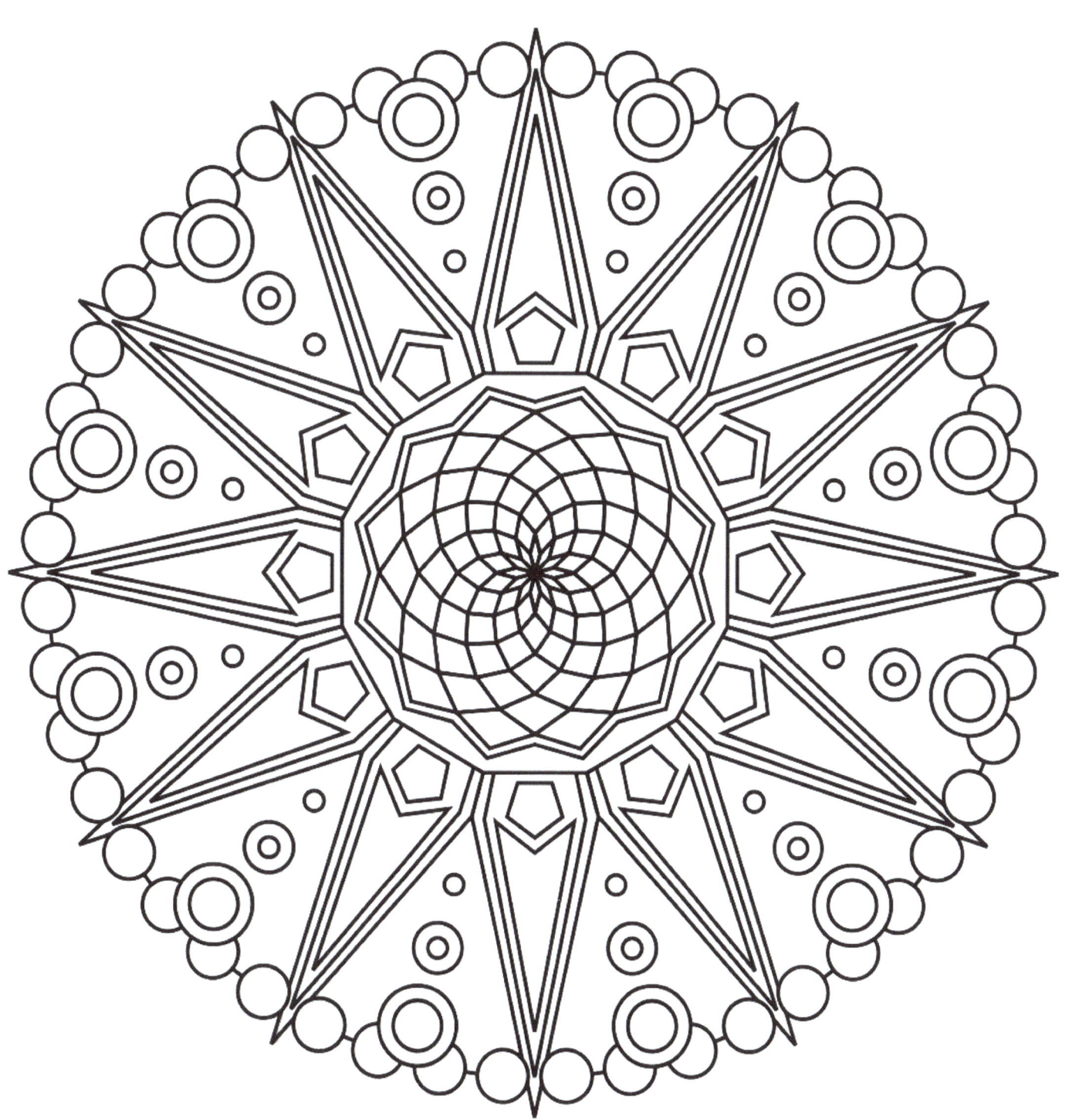

Step Four

Who Am I?

I made a searching and fearless moral inventory of myself - how am I contributing to the issue?

Willingness

Sometimes, we do things that don't really help out the situations that we are in. I can remember getting upset at my parent and either spouting something off full of attitude or slamming my door so hard that the house shook. However I chose to handle the situation, it was usually not the best way and it would set off a domino effect that would inevitably make the situation way bigger than it needed to be. Being in such a stressful environment, our minds go into defense mode and do what they think is necessary to protect us, which usually isn't always the best solution. I invite you to look deep into yourself to see in what ways you might make some situations worse with the way that you handle them.

Writing Directive

Take your own moral inventory. What have you done right? What have you done wrong? You are not perfect, and that's OK! Make a list of things that you would like to change about yourself. Try not to list physical things like being taller, or better at sports. Think deep inside and consider the negatives things you'd like to turn in to positive things.

___

"It is not the question, what am I going to be when I grow up; you should ask the question, who am I going to be when I grow up."
Goldie Hawn

Art Space

What does it feel like to see the negative parts of yourself? If these traits could come alive, (1) draw what would they look like? Now (2) write three positive statements about yourself use colors that describe how it feels when you think or say these positive statements.

Process What You Have Learned

How can you better the negative parts of yourself - through behaviors, feelings, or thoughts? Which positive statements will you begin using daily?

_____
_____
_____
_____
_____
_____
_____
_____
_____
_____
_____
_____
_____
_____
_____
_____
_____
_____
_____
_____
_____
_____
_____

Closing Artwork

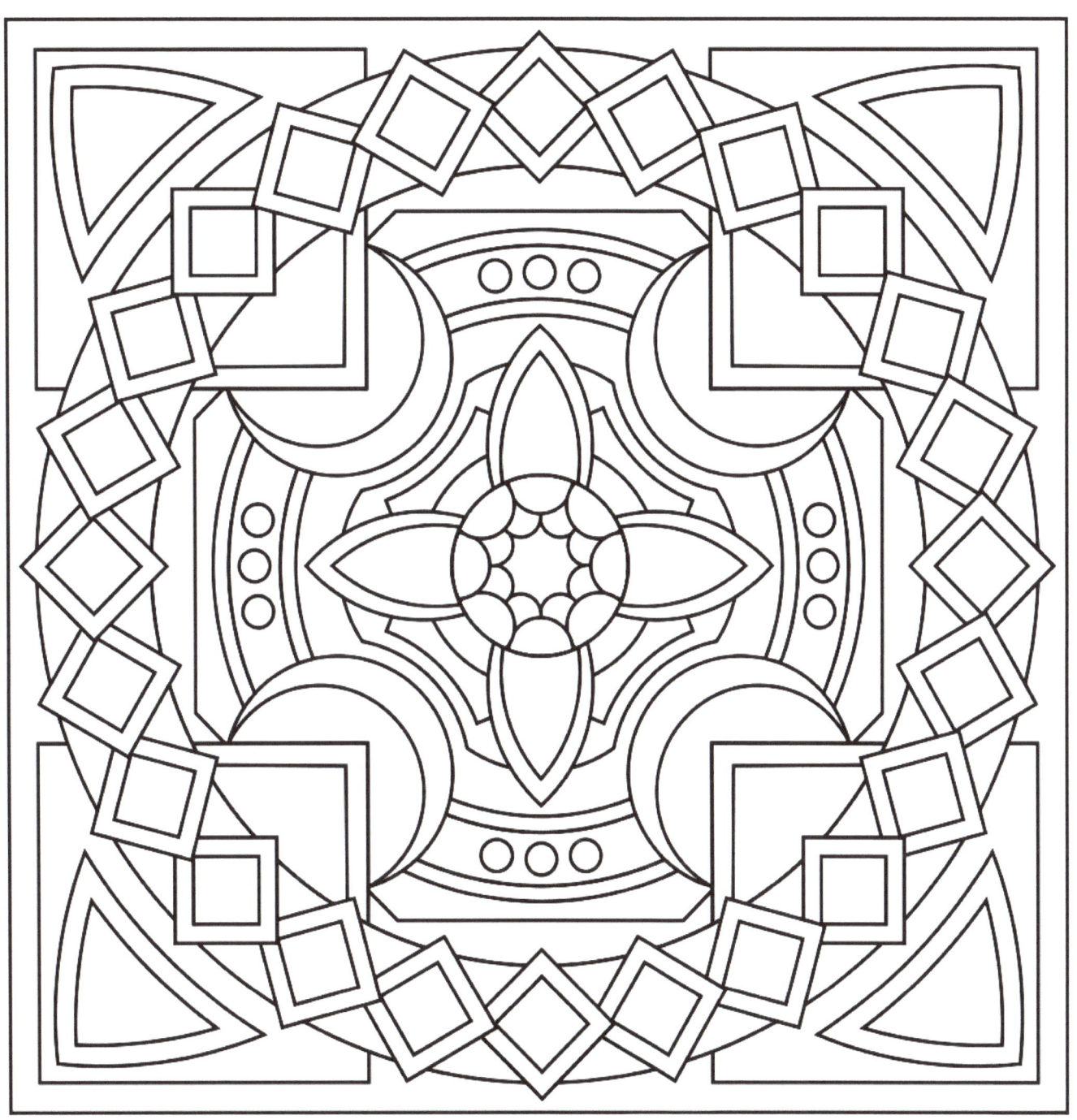

Step Five

I share who I am, with someone else

I admitted to myself and to another human being the exact nature of my situation

Integrity

There is nothing wrong with asking someone for their help. This shows integrity and strength rather than weakness. It takes a lot to admit that you cannot do something on your own - believe me I know. You have most likely spent most of your life trying to seem normal, put together, and strong. I can tell you from experience that after years of putting on the brave face it all eventually catches up with you. Imagine a soda bottle getting a good shake every once in a while. After some time that bottle is going to be more and more likely to explode the moment someone loosens the cap even just a little bit. No one wants to feel like a soda bottle. We all need help at some point in our lives and there is no shame in admitting that.

Writing Directive

Now it is time to reach out to the person that you trust. Pick a time, date, and place to meet up with this person (write it down) and use this section to plan out what you want to say. Sometimes meeting face to face can be scary, so you might want to start with writing a letter or talking on the phone first.

_____
_____
_____
_____
_____
_____
_____
_____
_____
_____
_____
_____
_____
_____
_____
_____
_____
_____
_____
_____
_____
_____
_____

"No one is useless in this world who lightens the burden
of it to anyone else."
Charles Dickens

Art Space

Draw what it was like to be in the meeting or to finish the meeting. What feelings were going on inside you at the time? Can you make an image showing this?

Process What You Have Learned

What did you notice or gain from sharing with someone? What do you still need?

Closing Artwork

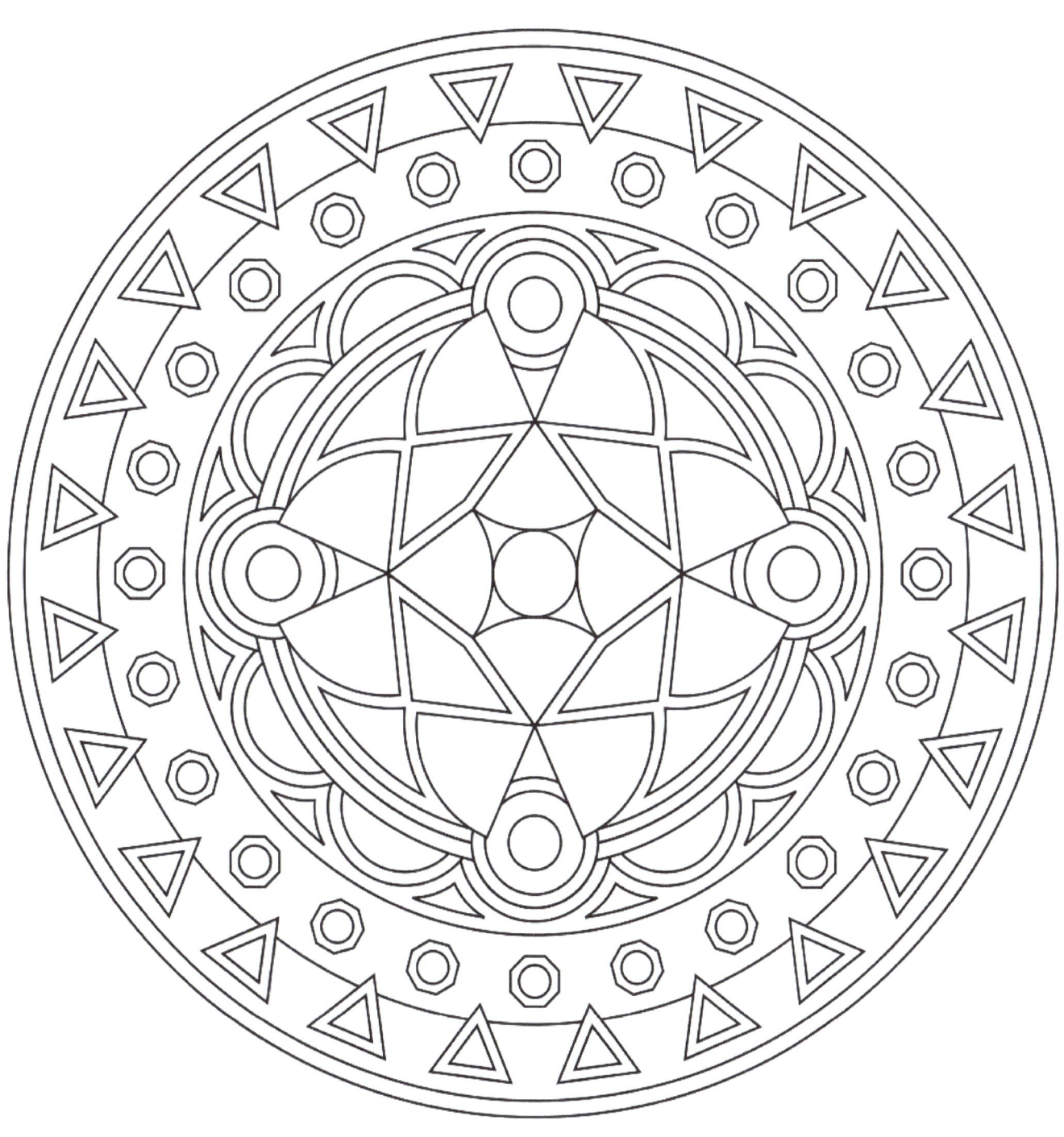

Step Six

Making Self Change

I am entirely ready to remove all defects of character and move forward in my life

Courage

You might feel like you have no courage at all, but think about how much courage it took to even pick up this book, to get all the way to step six. If it is still tough for you to feel courageous at this point, I completely understand, but celebrate your small victories. You have proven so much to yourself for making it this far, if to no one else, you have shown to yourself that you can handle any situation that you are faced with. Look back on all of the positive moves you have made so far and know that You Are Strong.

Writing Directive

Plan of action: Use this section to come back to when you need a reminder of all that you are accomplishing.

What do you need most today? _____
_____
_____

What do you need from family and friends? _____
_____
_____

What is your family member with mental illness capable of giving right now? _____
_____

Are these things realistic? _____
_____
_____

You are moving into adolescence and adulthood. What do YOU need to take care of yourself? _____
_____

What is going really well so far? _____
_____

How has your life changed? _____
_____
_____

Should I have another meeting with my trusted person to track my progress?

"You gain strength, courage, and confidence by every experience in which you really stop to look fear in the face. You are able to say to yourself, 'I lived through this horror. I can take the next thing that comes along.'"
Eleanor Roosevelt

Art Space

Make a storyboard (a comic strip) of different scenarios of conflict that happen often in your family and leave the ending blank. With what you have learned so far, think of better ways that you will handle these scenarios in the future and fill in the endings.

Process What You Have Learned

Describe the solutions that will most likely work and that you can realistically act upon in the future.

_____
_____
_____
_____
_____
_____
_____
_____
_____
_____
_____
_____
_____
_____
_____
_____
_____
_____
_____
_____
_____
_____
_____

Closing Artwork

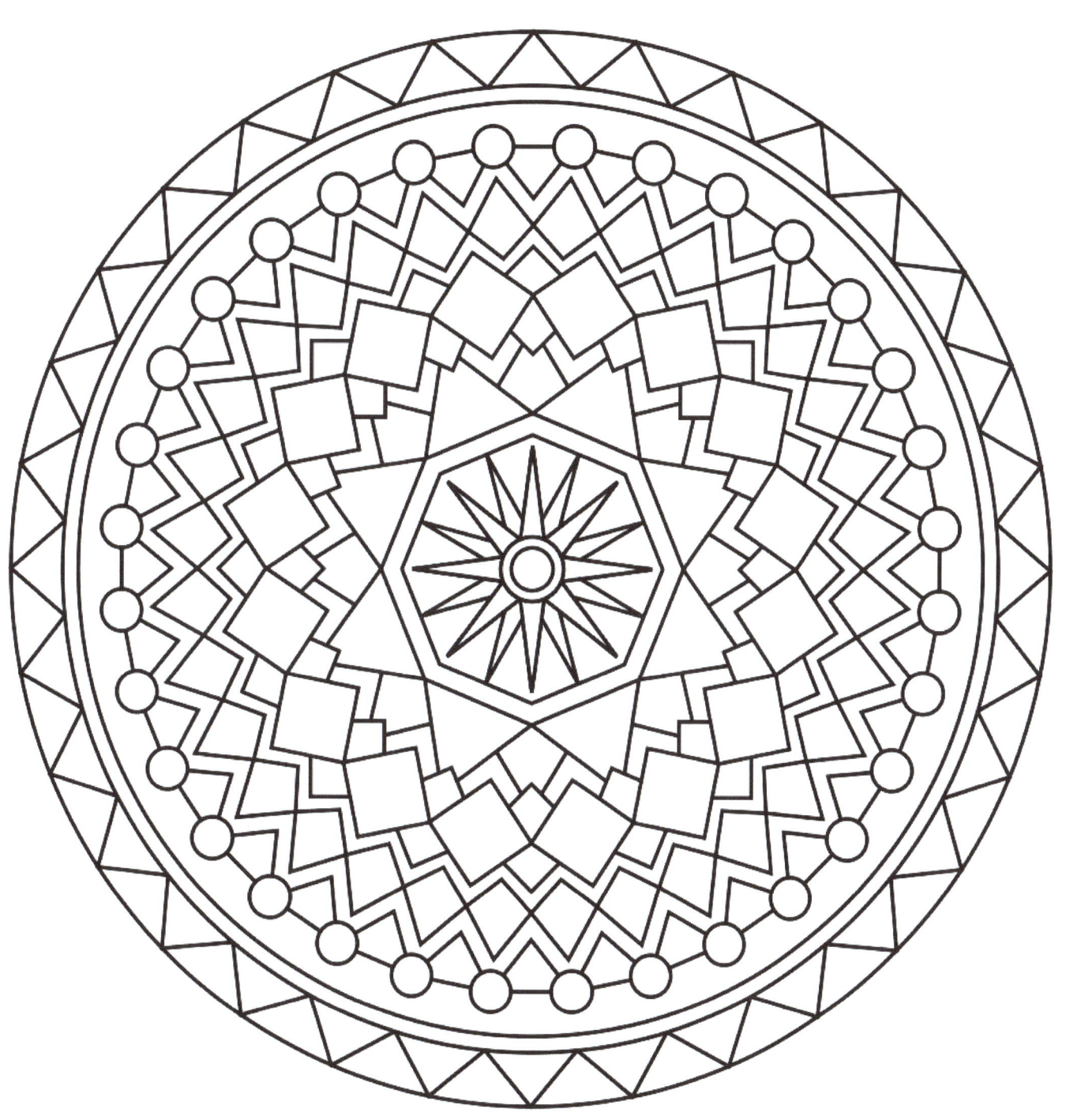

Step Seven

Start trying to change what I can!

I humbly ask for help to remove my shortcomings

Humility

You are not alone. Allow someone to help you carry your burden. Believe me, I spent almost 20 years trying to hide behind my fake strength, pretending to be okay, going along with how I was supposed to live life according to what all my friends were doing. Guess what? There are most likely things going on in your friends' lives that you don't know about as well. If you haven't come to a time in your life where you are exhausted from pretending for so long, you will, and when it happens, it is not going to be pretty. I used to climb into my bed and just crying for what seemed like forever. Every few months I would do this, get it all out, and go back to pretending everything was okay. Take it from someone who has been there... it is not fun. Be humble in the fact that you need help. Nothing says strength more than asking for help.

Writing Directive

Allow your trusted person to help you and give you someone to lean on to support you as you are developing into adulthood. You don't have to be tough all the time... let someone finally take some of the burden. In what ways do you most need help from someone else - someone to listen, to talk to, someone to give advice, or simply to spend time together etc.

_____
_____
_____
_____
_____
_____
_____
_____
_____
_____
_____
_____
_____
_____
_____
_____
_____
_____
_____
_____
_____

"Humility is always a good thing. It's always a good thing to be humbled by circumstances so you can then come from a sincere place to try to deal with them."
Michael J. Fox

Art Space

On these art pages, draw the burdens in a container that you have been carrying around by yourself for so long. Use a suitcase, bookbag, or any kind of container that you choose. Think about it busting at the seams from all of the extra weight that it can't support alone.

Art Space

Now use these two pages to draw an image of your trusted person helping relieve some of that burden for you.

Process What You Have Learned

Describe what it would be like to have some of your burden relieved:

_____
_____
_____
_____
_____
_____
_____
_____
_____
_____
_____
_____
_____
_____
_____
_____
_____
_____
_____
_____
_____
_____

Closing Artwork

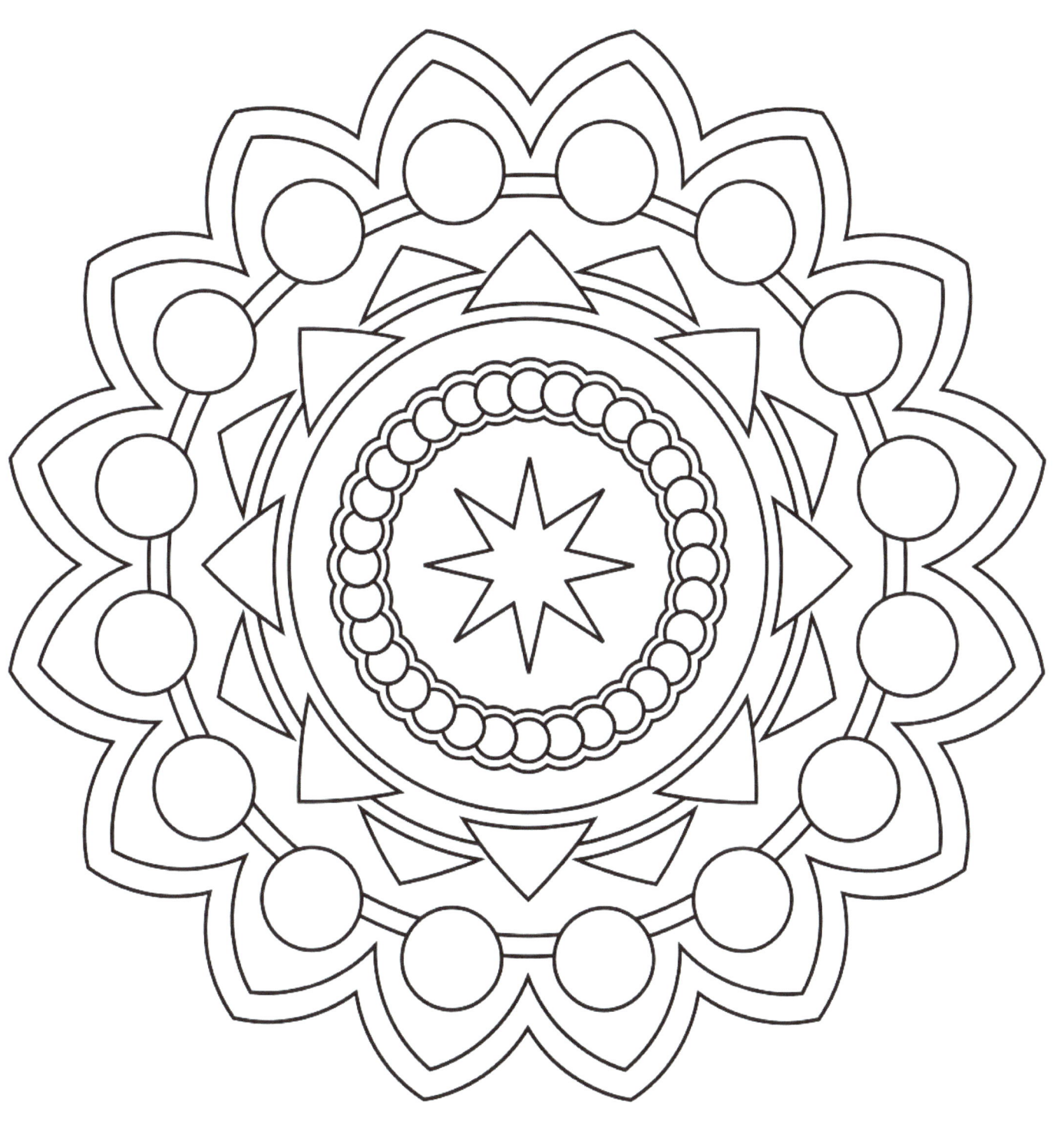

Step Eight

Make a list of the hurts that I have received from my family member

---

I made a list of all people who have hurt me, and become willing to make amends to them all

Compassion

This section may be one of the hardest of this book. How are you supposed to feel compassion for someone who has caused you so much pain over so many years? It is not easy, but it is possible. At some point in all of this, you are going to need to, at the least, begin looking at all of those hurts as strictly your family member's illness. I can almost guarantee that every interaction you have had with them has not been bad. Those positive times allow you to see just how much good they have inside of them. Have compassion for them as a person, their illness is something that they struggle with. It is not who they are.

Writing Directive

Make a list of the hurts that your caregiver has put onto you. How has each one made you feel?

_____
_____
_____
_____
_____
_____
_____
_____
_____
_____
_____
_____
_____
_____
_____
_____
_____
_____
_____
_____
_____
_____

"Grief can be the garden of compassion. If you keep your heart open through everything, your pain can become your greatest ally in your life's search for love and wisdom."
Rumi

Art Space

Assign a color to represent each 'hurt' and have an artistic conversation on the page. Answer those 'hurts' with positive statements about yourself, colors, or things you have learned from the workbook.

Process What You Have Learned

By recognizing the positive in my situation and developing compassion, I have learned:

_____
_____
_____
_____
_____
_____
_____
_____
_____
_____
_____
_____
_____
_____
_____
_____
_____
_____
_____
_____
_____
_____
_____
_____

Closing Artwork

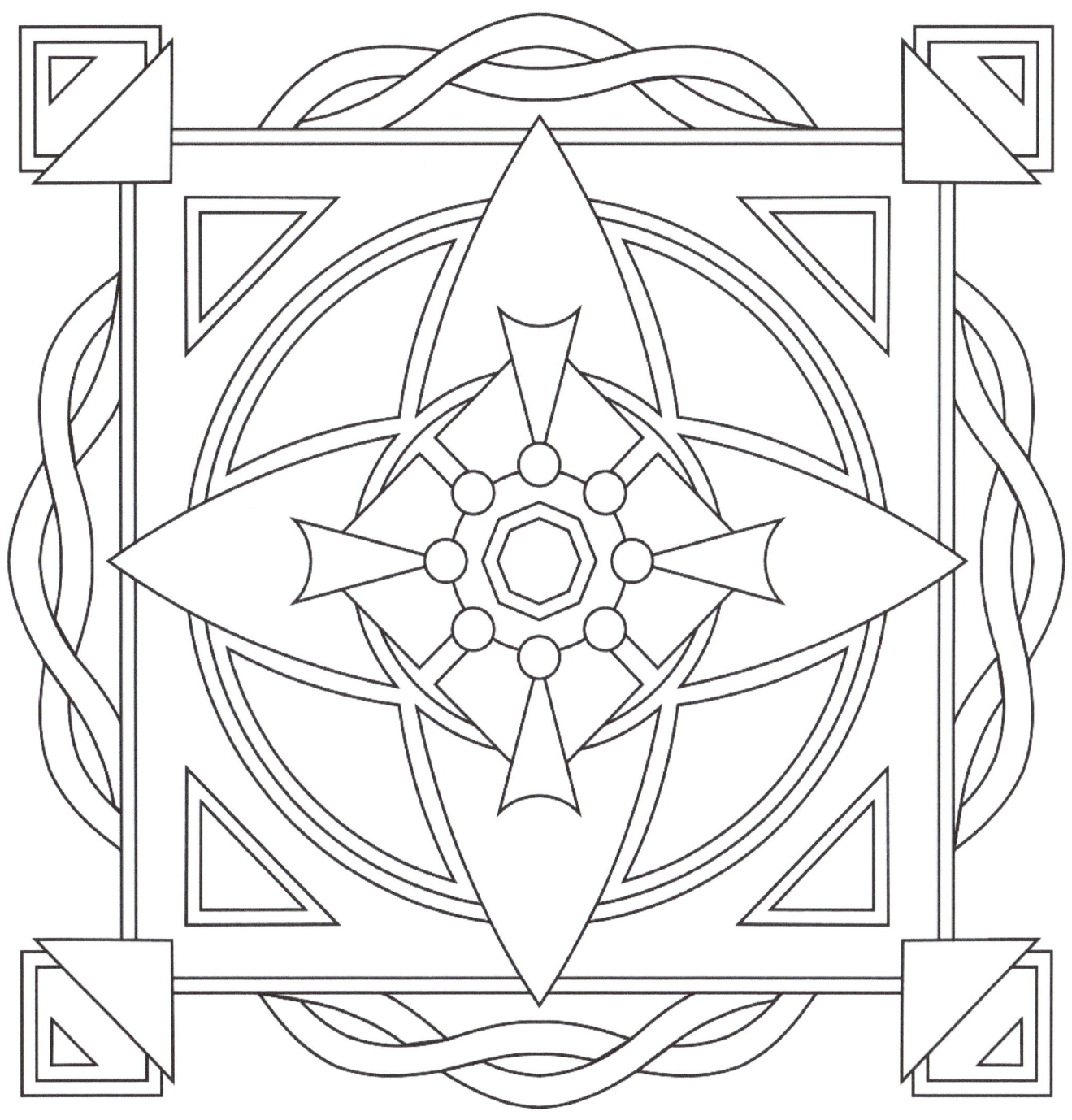

Step Nine

Mend things with that person

I made direct amends to such people whenever possible, except when to do so would injure them or others

Forgiveness

Let me be clear: forgiveness does not excuse anyone's actions towards you. That being said, forgiveness is more about you than anyone else. It allows you to be free of anger, guilt, and fear. Wouldn't it feel so great to not have to feel those things towards your family member anymore? I bet it is exhausting and heartbreaking to feel so negative all the time. Forgiveness allows you to be you again - it gives you the freedom to live your life again without always having to worry about the anger or guilt you feel. It's a great feeling to have the burden that you have been carrying around for so long suddenly lifted. It's almost as if you start to see things in a whole different way. Once the hate is out of your heart, the real healing can begin.

Writing Directive

Forgive, but don't forget. Write a pretend letter to your caregiver explaining how you felt throughout the 'situation'. (Remember: You do not need to send this letter; this is just for you as a part of letting go.)

Dear,

I forgive you for

_____

_____

_____

_____

_____

_____

_____

_____

_____

_____

_____

_____

_____

_____

_____

_____

_____

_____

"Forgiveness is the fragrance that the violet sheds on the heel that has crushed it."
Mark Twain

Art Space

1. First, draw random lines or squiggles that cross and intersect
2. Choose what pattern or designs you want to use
3. Fill the sections with different patterns or designs

Examples of patterns:

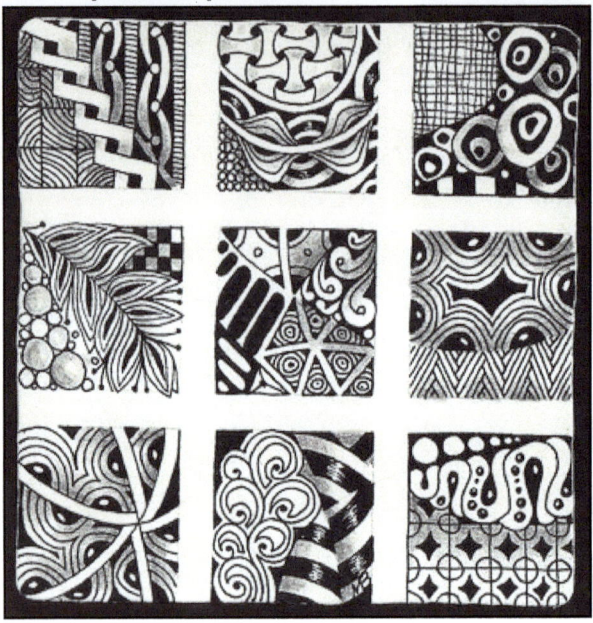

Insert your patterns:

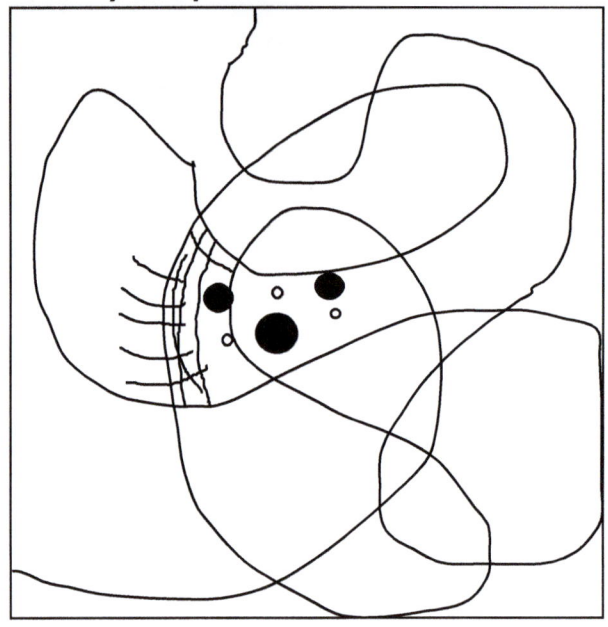

Insert your patterns:

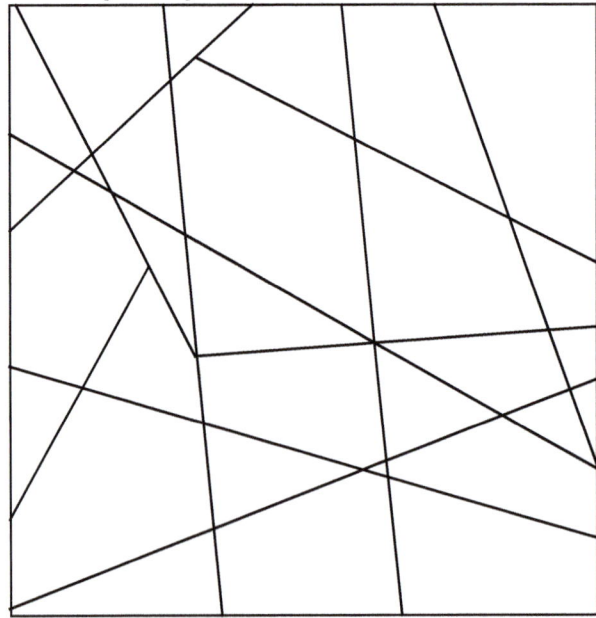

"One of the lovely things about Zentangle is that it isn't supposed to BE anything. Even more, it's SUPPOSED to NOT be a something. ... Zentangle is simply beautiful patterns playing harmoniously together." - Margaret Bramner

You probably have a lot of different emotions running through your mind after that last writing directive. On these two art pages, I have provided you with zentangles to help you calm down. When you feel up to continuing, move on to the next two art pages.

Now you try...

How do you feel after Zentangling....

_____
_____
_____
_____

Art Space

Now, make an image representing how you think making amends with the person that hurt you would go.

Process What You Have Learned

What are the benefits and challanges of making amends?

Closing Artwork

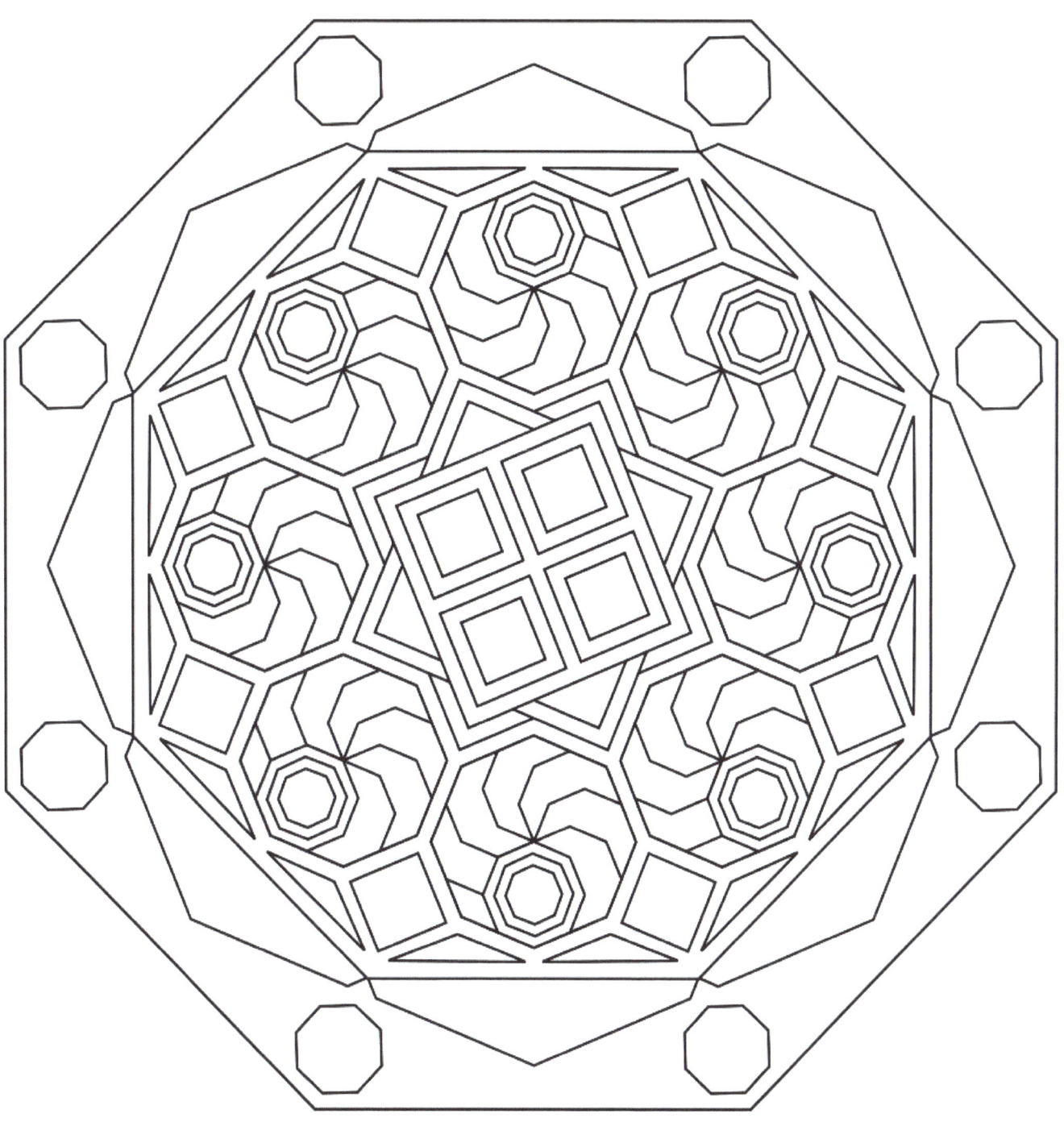

Step Ten

How am I doing?

I continued to take personal inventory and when I was wrong, I promptly admitted it.

Perseverance

You have come so far, and you should be so proud of yourself! You have pushed through and made yourself face some pretty difficult things. Now is not the time to give up. Keep pushing and allow yourself to finally feel better. Many people would have stopped by now, saying that it was too hard, or that they weren't ready, but you aren't one of them. You are strong and you have proven to yourself that you can handle anything from now on. You have grown so much throughout this workbook and you should be proud of yourself.

Writing Directive

Weekly "come back to" page. Review steps one through nine and think about the progress you have made so far. If you feel yourself slipping or sliding backwards, start back at step one and compare your new answers to your old ones. List what you've learned or how this has helped you so far. Write anything down that is not working and go back to the step that matches your concern.

___

"A hero is an ordinary individual who finds the strength to persevere and endure in spite of overwhelming obstacles."
Christopher Reeve

Art Space

Are you experiencing any current distress or tension? Draw an outline of your body. Use color to represent where you feel tension and what it feels like, and add it to the body.

Process What You Have Learned

Now that you see where you are feeling most of your tension/distress, what can you do to relieve it? Which step can you look back at, to help you continue to grow?

_____
_____
_____
_____
_____
_____
_____
_____
_____
_____
_____
_____
_____
_____
_____
_____
_____
_____
_____
_____
_____
_____

Closing Artwork

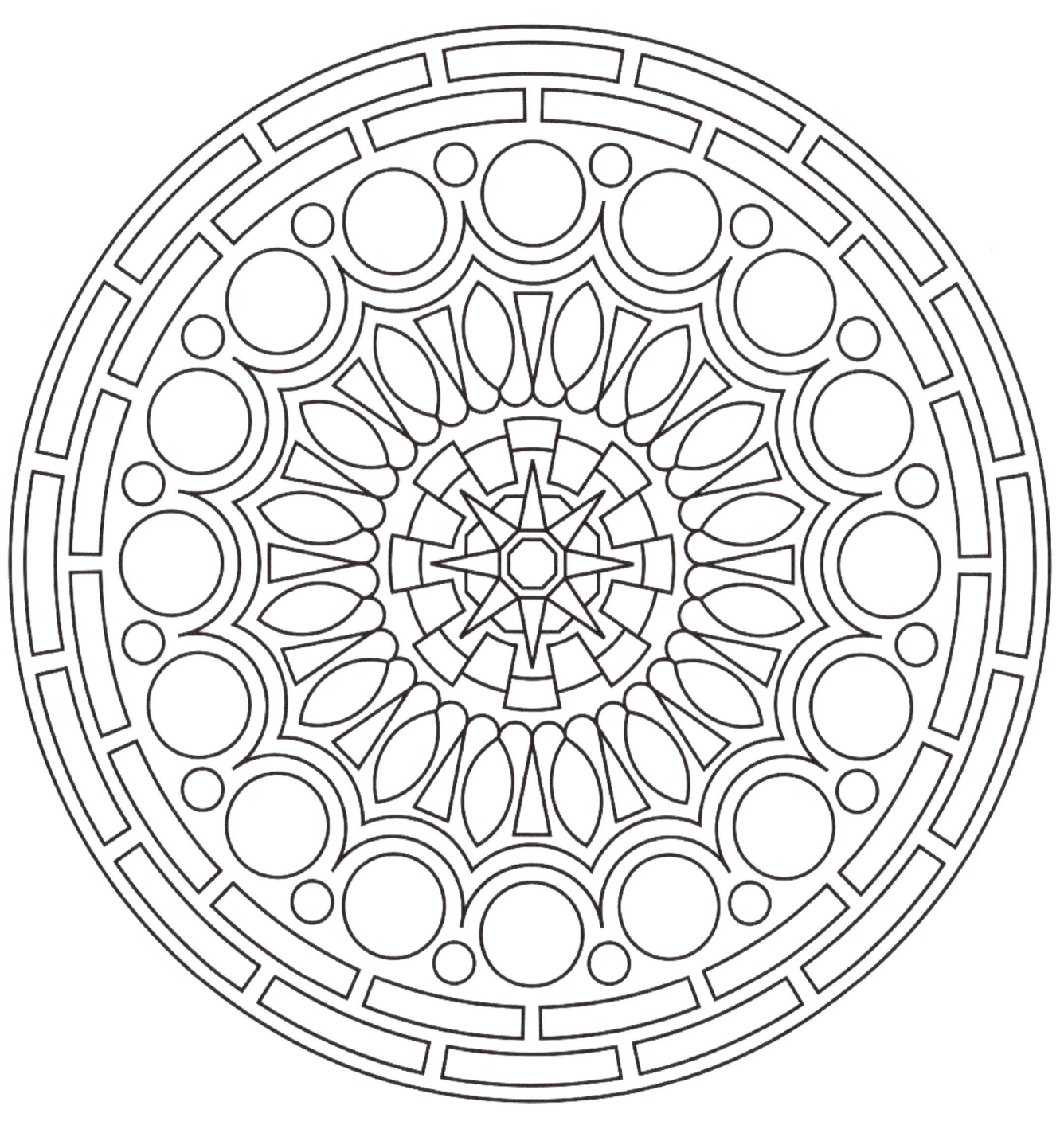

Step Eleven

Continue to grow daily!

I have sought self-awareness to improve my understanding of my situation and the situation itself, and seek the knowledge and the power to carry out what I have learned so far.

Self - Awareness

It is important to remind yourself every day what you have learned, what you are doing, and why you are doing it. Be aware how certain situations make you feel and use these steps to plan the most successful route of action. You are the only one who can control how you handle situations. You cannot always control how someone else acts, but it is entirely in your power to decide how you are going to react.

Writing Directive

Who is in control of me? ME. Only I can change me. No matter how bad a 'situation' is, I will always have some sort of choice. Use this check-list to make sure that you are on track and are completing the things that should be in your life by now:

Have I been honest with myself? How?
_____
_____
_____

Do I have a more positive attitude than before starting this book?
_____
_____
_____

How are my relationships with other members of my family different?
_____
_____

In what ways have I allowed my trusted person to take some of my burden?
_____
_____

How has forgiveness of my family member altered our relationship?
_____
_____

If any of your answers do not live up to your expectations, please feel free to flip back to that chapter of the book and see what you need to do differently.

"People need to know that they have all the tools within themselves. Self-awareness, which means awareness of their body, awareness of their mental space, awareness of their relationships - not only with each other, but with life and the ecosystem."
Deepak Chopra

Art Space

Think about the first art piece you did in this workbook, the road map. Keeping that in mind, I would like for you to draw your life in regard to two different pathways: the Positive Path and the Negative Path. Consider what makes one positive and the other negative.

Process What You Have Learned

What path are you on at this very moment? If it is still the Negative Path, what do you need to do to get onto the Positive Path?

_____
_____
_____
_____
_____
_____
_____
_____
_____
_____
_____
_____
_____
_____
_____
_____
_____
_____
_____
_____
_____
_____
_____
_____

Closing Artwork

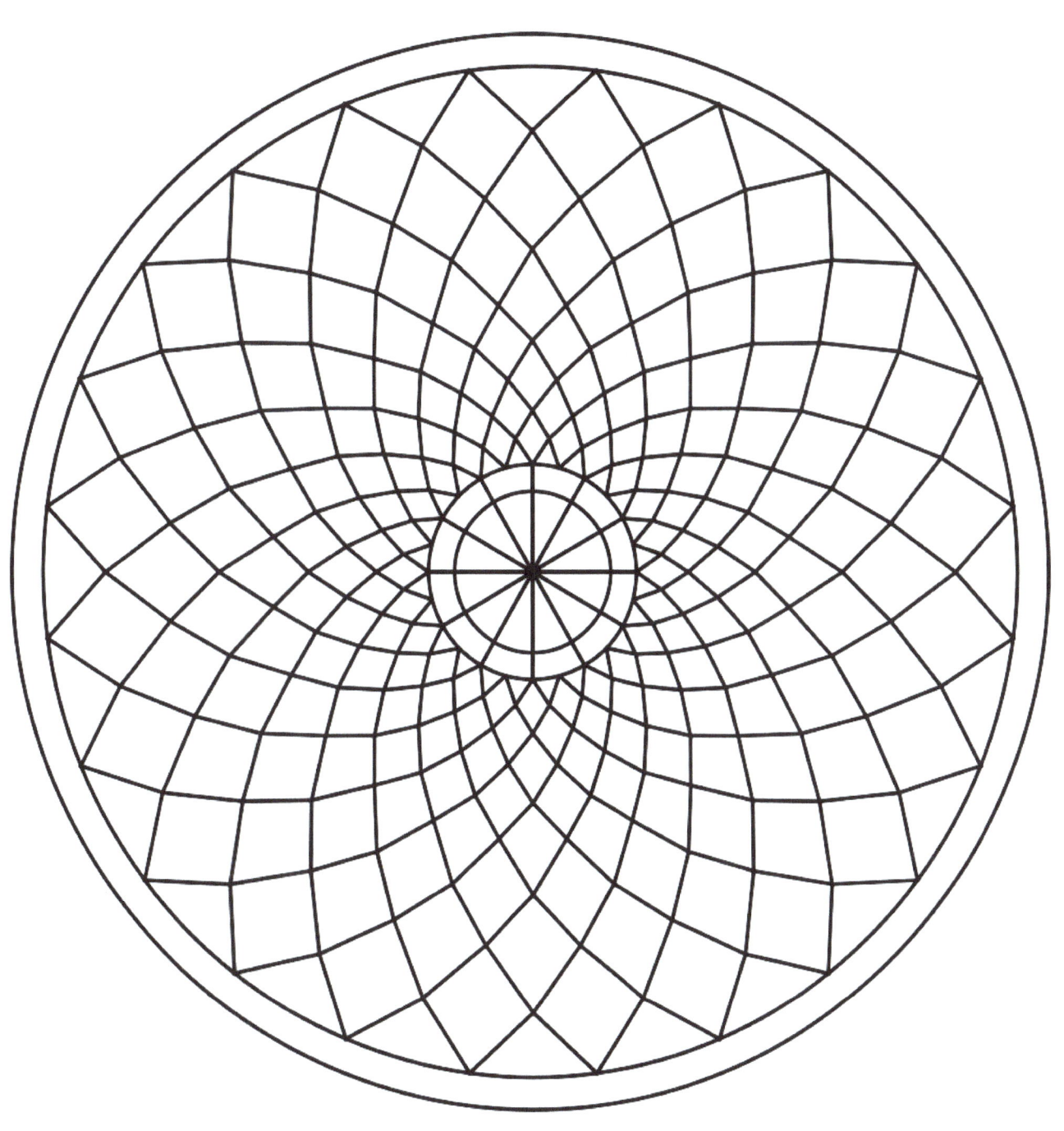

Step Twelve

Try to practice what I have learned

I have had a self-awakening as the result of these steps, I have tried to carry this message to othes in my situation, and I have practiced these principles in all of my life affairs

Service to Others

With everything that you have learned, why wouldn't you want to reach out and help someone else who may be in the same situation? In the best case scenario, you may not know anyone specifically who you believe to be in some kind of turmoil, but at least your own experiences can prepare you for when you do. If nothing else, this workbook has allowed you to see that you are not alone - there are others who may be suffering - and you now have the knowledge to help them.

Writing Directive

Do you know anyone else struggling with a "situation"? How can you become the trusted person that helped you? How can you help others get stronger, and get them on the Positive Path?

_____
_____
_____
_____
_____
_____
_____
_____
_____
_____
_____
_____
_____
_____
_____
_____
_____
_____
_____
_____
_____
_____

"To lose yourself in righteous service to others can lift your sights and get your mind off personal problems, or at least put them in proper focus."
Ezra Taft Benson

Art Space

Pretend that you live in a community where the other adolescents are in your same "situation". If money was no object, what kind of community would you build to help support these adolescents? What kinds of services would you offer or places would you provide? Use symbols to draw the community.

Process What You Have Learned

What does it feel like to be done with this process? What are your thoughts, feelings, or ideas about moving forward from this point on?

_____
_____
_____
_____
_____
_____
_____
_____
_____
_____
_____
_____
_____
_____
_____
_____
_____
_____
_____
_____
_____
_____
_____
_____
_____

Congratulations!

You've completed the 12 Steps to coping with a parent/guardian who has a mental illness. Complete the following statement:

I cope with my _____ who has a mental illness of _____

by (list ways that you have learned to cope) _____

_____

_____

_____

I can lean on _____ for support. And I know _____'s

illness is about them, and not about me. I am (Your positive self statements) _____

_____

_____

and in the future I will _____.

Meet Your Author

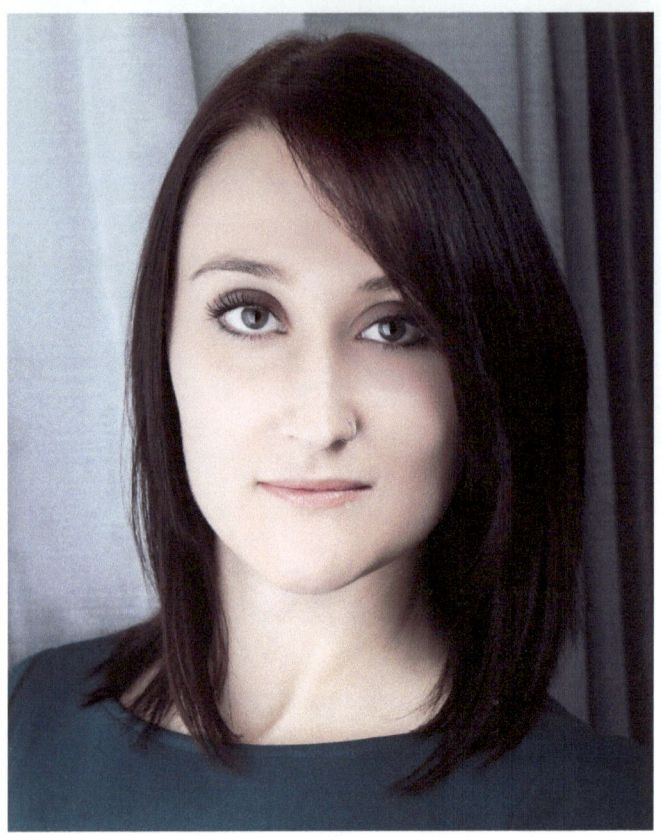

I was born in a small Southwestern Virginia town where I attended a vocational art school in conjunction with high school. Each morning from zero to first period, I would spend that time doing art, and then head back to finish out my school day. It was at this vocational school that I fell in love with the idea of pursuing art as a career. Unfortunately, my lack of confidence told me that fine art was most likely not going to pay the bills, so I needed to find a major in college. I decided to enroll in the Graphic Design program at Longwood University in Farmville, VA, in hopes of graduating to work as a graphic designer in new business branding. I wanted to get a great job that would take me far away - far from the home life that I had grown up in.

Things weren't always rainbows and sunshine at home. I lived in what I would later learn was a 'toxic environment' and was left to cope with the situation on my own. My mother was always critical of anything that could be criticized, while my father was usually mentally 'checked-out'. Their relationship in general was toxic. Screaming, threatening, things getting broken and holes being put into the walls, this combination didn't lead me to invite many school friends over for sleepovers. These situations left me feeling that the one place that was supposed to be safe, home, was not. These were the times that I sat behind a locked bedroom door and sketched. I was a kid. I didn't do everything right and I didn't always have the best attitude, so I never knew if what I was going to say or do was going to start World War III. I walked through the halls of my high school looking at the happy, smiling kids assuming that their lives at home were perfect. It was exhausting trying to hide my secret from everyone. Constantly going to other peoples houses, and avoiding the questions of why they could never come over to mine , led me to pull back and always find excuses to not hang out with friends outside of school…
Eventually the invitations stopped all together.

In the tenth grade, the fight to end all fights ensued leaving my dad to move to a hotel, my mom in a crumpled mess on their bedroom floor blaming me, and my younger brother and I to become the parents. I became the messenger, the sounding board, the confidant, and the therapist to each of my parents separately.

I was forced to become an adult before I could even legally drive. I was inadvertently asked to take care of my parents' marriage. Somewhere in my senior year of college, I began to play with the idea of tossing all of the graphic design schooling to the wind and becoming a therapist; I already had a lot of practice. One of my classmates had begun talking about a graduate program in art therapy that she was going to attend and it sparked my interest. Maybe I could become a therapist after all, without having to give up the one thing that had gotten me through all of those years at home - the artwork.

In 2014, I graduated from Longwood University with a Bachelor's degree in Graphic Design and immediately that fall was enrolled in the Graduate Art Therapy and Counseling program at Eastern Virginia Medical School. It was there that I had finally found the one thing that allowed me to feel passion and confidence in life - helping people through the use of art. It is my hope that this book, the only one of its kind, will give young boys and girls the skills and support that I myself did not receive.
If but only one child is helped by this workbook and my testimony to the healing properties of art, then my hard work and dedication was worth something.

> "Behind every creative adult, there is a child that survived."
> - anonymous

Need More Resources?

Try These:

www.Arttherapy.org

www.Enthusiasticartist.blogspot.com

www.Creative12steps.blogspot.com

www.Printmadala.com

www.Al-anon.org

www.mentalhealth4kids.org

www.suicidepreventionlifeline.org

References

Al-Anon Family Group Headquarters, Inc. (n.d.). Welcome to Al-Anon Family Groups. (n.d.). Retrieved from http://al-anon.org/

Aldridge, J., & Sharpe, D. (2009). Pictures of young caring. Criminal Justice Matters, 78(1), 38-40. doi:10.1080/09627250903385289

American Psychiatric Association. (1994). Diagnostic and statistical manual of mental disorders (4th ed.). Washington, D.C: Author.

American Psychiatric Association. (2013). Diagnostic and statistical manual of mental disorders (5th ed.). Washington, D.C: Author.

Bartsch, D., Roberts, R., Davies, M., & Proeve, M. (2014). The impact of parental diagnosis of borderline personality disorder on offspring: Learning from clinical practice. Personality and Mental Health, 9, 33-43. doi: 10.1002/pmh.1274

Beck, J. S. (2011). Cognitive behavior therapy: Basics and beyond (2nd ed.). New York: The Guilford Press.

Berg-Nielsen, T., & Wichstrom, L. (2012). The mental health of preschoolers in a Norwegian population-based study when their parents have symptoms of borderline, antisocial, and narcissistic personality disorders: At the mercy of unpredictability. Child and Adolescent Psychiatry and Mental Health, 6(1), 19

Bremner, M. (n.d.). Enthusiastic artist [Blog post]. Retrieved from http://enthusiasticartist.blogspot.com/

Chamberlin, J. (2004). Survey says: More Americans are seeking mental health treatment. Monitor on Psychology, 35(7), 17.

Coping skill. (2009). Medical dictionary. Retrieved from http://medical-dictionary.thefreedictionary.com/coping+skill

Creative guide through the 12 steps/ (n.d.). Retrieved from http://creative 12steps.blogspot.com/

Curry, N., & Kasser, T. (2005): Can coloring mandalas reduce anxiety? Art Therapy: Journal of the American Art Therapy Association, 22(2), 81-85.

Deaver, S., & McAuliffe, G. (2009). Reflective visual journaling during art therapy and counseling internships: A qualitative study. Reflective Practice, 10(5), 615-632.

Farmer, L. (2010). Zentangles. Retrieved March 11, 2016, from http://tanglepatterns.com/zentangles

Fraser, E., & Pakenham, K. I. (2008). Evaluation of a resilience-based intervention for children of parents with mental illness. Australian & New Zealand Journal of Psychiatry, 42(12), 1041-1050. doi:10.1080/00048670802512065

Fraser, E., & Pakenham, K. I. (2009). Resilience in children of parents with mental illness: Relations between mental health literacy, social connectedness and coping, and both adjustment and caregiving. Psychology, Health & Medicine, 14(5), 573-584. doi:10.1080/13548500903193820

Goodyear, M., Cuff, R., Maybery, D., & Reupert, A. (2009). CHAMPS: A peer support program for children of parents with a mental illness. Advances in Mental Health, 8(3), 296-304. doi:10.5172/jamh.8.3.296

Hancock, K. J., Mitrou, F., Shipley, M., Lawrence, D., & Zubrick, S. R. (2013). A three generation study of the mental health relationships between grandparents, parents and children. BMC Psychiatry, 13(1), 299. doi:10.1186/1471-244x-13-299

Hargreaves, J., Bond, L., O'Brien, M., Forer, D., & Davies, L. (2008). The PATS peer support program: Prevention/early intervention for adolescents who have a parent with mental illness. Youth Studies Australia, 27(1), 43-51.

Hinden, B. R., Biebel, K., Nicholson, J., & Mehnert, L. (2005). The invisible children's project: Key ingredients of an intervention for parents with mental illness. Journal of Behavioral Health Services & Resesarch, 32(4), 393-408.

Hinden, B.R., Biebel, K., Nicholson, J., Henry, A., & Stier, L. (2002). Steps toward evidence-based practices for parents with mental illness and their families. Rockville, MD: Substance Abuse and Mental Health Services Administration.

Hinz, L. D. (2009). Expressive Therapies Continuum: A framework for using art in therapy. New York: Routledge.

Homlong, L., Rosvold, E. O., Sagatun, Å., Wentzel-Larsen, T., & Haavet, O. R. (2015). Living with mentally ill parents during adolescence: A risk factor for future welfare dependence? A longitudinal, population-based study. BMC Public Health, 15(1), 413. doi:10.1186/s12889-015-1734-1

Humphreys, K. (1996). World view change in adult children of Alcoholics/Al-Anon self-help groups: Reconstructing the alcoholic family. International Journal of of Group Psychotherapy, 46(2), 255-263.

Ireland, M. J., & Pakenham, K. I. (2010). Youth adjustment to parental illness or disability: The role of illness characteristics, caregiving, and attachment. Psychology, Health & Medicine, 15(6), 632-645. doi:10.1080/13548506.2010.498891

Julliard, K. (1999). The twelve steps and art therapy. Mundelein, IL: American Art Therapy Association.

Krebs, K. A. (2008). Art therapy used to enhance steps one, two and three of a twelve-step recovery program for addictions treatment (Unpublished master's thesis) Ursuline College, Pepper Pike, OH.

Lagacá-Ságuin, D., & Gionet, A. (2012). Parental meta-emotion and temperament predict coping skills in early adolescence. International Journal of Adolescence and Youth, 14(4), 367-382.

Lounsbury. (2014). Art therapy to support recovery from substance use disorders (Master's thesis). Retrieved from http://alfredadler.edu/library/masters/2014/lisa-marie-lounsbury

Lyshack-Stelzer, F., Singer, P., St. John, P., & Chemtob, C. (2007). Art therapy for adolescents with posttraumatic stress disorder symptoms: A pilot study. Art Therapy: Journal of the American Art Therapy Association, 24(4), 163-169.

Macfie, J. (2009). Development in children and adolescents whose mothers have borderline personality disorder. Child Development Perspectives, 3, 66-71.

Marsh, D. (2000). Children of parents with mental illness. Retrieved from https://www.bccf.ca/bccf/resources/children-of-parents-with-mental-illness/

Marston, N., Maybery, D., & Reupert, A. (2014). Empowering families where a parent has a mental illness: A preliminary evaluation of the "Family Focus" DVD. Advances in Mental Health, 12(2), 136-146. doi:10.5172/jamh.2013.4679

Meichenbaum, D. (1977). Cognitive behaviour modification. Scandinavian Journal of Behaviour Therapy, 6(4), 185-192. doi:10.1080/16506073.1977.9626708

Mental Health America of Hawaii (n.d.). Some parents with mental illness have families [PDF document]. Retrieved from http://www.mentalhealthhi.org/Resources/Documents/invisible%20children%20power%20point.pdf

Murphy, G., Peters, K., Jackson, D., & Wilkes, L. (2011). A qualitative meta-synthesis of adult children of parents with a mental illness. Journal of Clinical Nursing, 20(23-24), 3430-3442. doi:10.1111/j.1365-2702.2010.03651.x

Ola, B., Suren, R., & Ani, C. (2015). Depressive symptoms among children whose parents have serious mental illness: Association with children's threat-related beliefs about mental illness. South African Journal of Psychiatry, 21(3), 74-78. doi:10.7196/sajp.8253

Sandmire, D., Gorham, S., Rankin, N., & Grimm, D. (2012). The influence of art making on anxiety: A pilot study. Art Therapy: Journal of the American Art Therapy Association, 29(2), 68-73.

Shor, R., Kalivatz, Z., Amir, Y., Aldor, R., & Lipot, M. (2014). Therapeutic factors in a group for parents with mental illness. Community Mental Health Journal, 51(1), 79-84. doi:10.1007/s10597-014-9739-2

Spier, E. (2010). Group art therapy with eighth-grade students transitioning to high school. Art Therapy: Journal of the American Art Therapy Association, 27(2), 75-83. doi: 10.1080/07421656.2010.10129717

Stoeckel, M., Weissbrod. C., & Ahrens, A. (2014). The adolescent response to parental illness: The influence of dispositional gratitude. Journal of Child and Family Studies, 24(5), 1501-1509

The 12 Steps. (n.d.). Retrieved from http://www.12step.org/the-12-steps

Tussing, H. L., & Valentine, D. P. (2001). Helping adolescents cope with the mental illness of a parent though bibliotherapy. Child and Adolescent Social Work Journal, 18(6), 455-469.

Van Lith, T. (2015). Art making as a mental health recovery tool for change and coping. Art Therapy: Journal of the American Art Therapy Association, 32(1), 5-12.

Van Loon, L. M., Van de Ven, M. O., Van Doesum, K. T., Witteman, C. L., & Hosman, C. M. (2013). The relation between parental mental illness and adolescent mental health: The role of family factors. Journal of Child and Family Studies, 23(7), 1201-1214. doi:10.1007/s10826-013-9781-7

Versions of the 12 Steps from Different Fellowships. (n.d.). Retrieved from http://www.12step.org/references/12-step-versions/

Vimont, C. (2009). Adapting 12 step programs for teenagers. Retrieved from http://12wisdomsteps.com/NewAdditions/Adapting12StepProgramsforTeenagers.html

Wansink, H., Janssens, J., Hoencamp, E., Middelkoop, B., & Hosman, C. (2015). Effects of preventative family service coordination for parents with mental illnesses and their children, a RCT. Families, Systems, & Health, 33(2), 110-119.

www.ingramcontent.com/pod-product-compliance
Lightning Source LLC
Chambersburg PA
CBHW051156220526
45473CB00003B/797